KETOGENIC DIET FOR BEGINNERS

MUST KNOW - DO'S AND DON'TS FOR BEGINNERS

TABLE OF CONTENTS

INTRODUCTION

Your health is something that is personal and this means that what could be your meat could be another's poison. Furthermore, there are selected health rules that have been proven to be beneficial on this type of effective diet. This book will offer you with all the information you need to know on how to begin the keto diet, what foods to eat, the ones to avoid, meal plans as well as the recipes you can follow while on this diet.

This ketogenic diet book will act as a resource for you in knowing everything about the low-carb diet. It will cover the psychology behind such diets, including potential negative effects as well as giving specific recommendations on how to optimize such a diet.

Have no worries in case you were searching for the best keto book to assist you master a low carb diet. Your search stops here; so don't dare put this book down. Diets that are low in carbs are not quite new in the weight-loss scene.

Do you regard a low-carb diet simply as a way of losing weight? What if you discovered that when you combine a low-carb diet with high fat intake, you will produce a powerful effect on a wide variety of health conditions?

The Ketogenic diet is one of the most popular diets in the world of weight loss right now for many reasons. Thousands have enjoyed the many health benefits including lower blood pressure, lower cholesterol, more energy, clearer thinking, and of course weight loss. Many also believe and follow the ketogenic diet to fight cancer as well. The ketogenic diet allows you to eat real foods, the ones you are already used to eating, and you will still lose the weight you want to lose. Using proven methods to help your body and metabolism work together, you will lose weight in your sleep!

This guide teaches you all about the Ketogenic Diet basics and how you can use this fast weight loss eating plan to your body to use fat storage as energy first, while guiding you step by step towards a healthier lifestyle.

This book contains recipes, benefits and proven ways of benefitting from the Ketogenic diet. It details the health benefits of this diet and ways of starting and maintaining it.

In the 1920s and on to the 30s, the keto diet's popularity soared as an epilepsy therapy. Since fasting had been successfully used as a therapy for epileptics, the Ketogenic diet was introduced as an alternative to mainstream fasting. However, as the years passed, this diet was done away with because new anti-convulsion therapies had been introduced. After it was realized that the medication still failed to achieve the desired control in around 25% of the sufferers, the keto diet was re-introduced especially among kids.

In 1921, Woodyatt made two important observations; acetone and beta-hydroxybutyric acid appear in a normal subject through starvation or a diet that has low levels of carbs and a lot of fat. At the same time, Dr. Wilder of the Mayo clinic proposed that a Keto diet be tried as a therapy for epileptics. He was of the view that the diet had to be as effective as fasting, but could be maintained for a longer span of time. As a result, Wilder supervised on patients treated with the ketone-producing diet at the Mayo clinic and he came up with the term, "ketogenic diet".

Further, Peterman of the Mayo clinic reported the ratio of ketogenic diets the same as the ones used today; 1g of protein per kg of body weight in children, 10-5g of carbs on a daily basis, and the remainder of calories in fat. This was in 1925. He also recorded the usefulness of caregivers being taught the management of the keto diet before discharge and close follow-up. Peterman also noted behavior and cognitive improvements that came with the ketogenic diet. His reports were quickly followed by reports from Talbot et al. from Harvard and McQuarrie and Keith, also from the Mayo clinic.

The utilization of the keto diet was documented in many books that discussed epilepsy in children, between 1941 and 1980. A large number of these books described the diet, how to start it as well as the diet plans. In the year 1972, Livingston, from John Hopkins Hospital studied the effect of the diet in over 1,000 epileptic kids. He reported that 52% of the children were able to control their seizures and an extra 20% had improved control.

But when the ketogenic diet therapy was ignored, fewer dieticians were trained on this diet and a shortage resulted. This resulted in the implantation of the ketogenic diet without proper calculation, leading to the public perception that the diet was not effective. Consequently, this diet has always relied on public perception.

However, in the recent past, the keto diet has experienced resurgence. This diet is now practiced in over 45 countries even though the perception of physicians still greatly affects the utilization of this therapy by pediatric neurologists. There are two surveys; one was done in America and the other in Europe. The surveys found out that the ketogenic diet was the last alternative form of treatment in almost all childhood epilepsies.

Understanding the ketogenic diet

In this diet, you need to know that ketosis is the unique feature. The keto diet is high in fat, offers enough protein and is low in carbs. This combination alters the manner in which energy is utilized by the body. Fat is converted in the liver into fatty acids and ketone bodies. Another effect of this diet is that it lowers the levels of glucose and enhances the resistance of insulin.

The keto diet is also effective when it comes to losing weight and improving your overall health. It has benefits when it comes to fighting diabetes, cancer, epilepsy and Alzheimer's disease. Also, this diet has similarities the Atkins as well as other low-carb diets. It involves drastically cutting down on carbs and substituting it with fat. This reduction in carbohydrate intake places the body in a state of metabolism known as ketosis. When in ketosis, your body will be efficient in burning fat to release energy. Moreover, fat is also turned into ketones in the liver, and the brain can be supplied with energy.

Metabolic syndrome

It involves the grouping of at least three out of five of the following medical conditions:

1. High blood pressure
2. Low high density lipoprotein levels
3. High serum triglycerides
4. High blood glucose
5. Abdominal or central obesity

Having just one of the above conditions does not mean that you are suffering from metabolic syndrome. Having more than one of them increases the risk. Metabolic syndrome increases the risk of having cardiovascular ailments and diabetes.

Research has shown that the prevalence in America is at an estimated thirty percent of the adult population. Furthermore, the prevalence increases with age. This syndrome and pre diabetes have similarities but are diagnosed with different biomarkers.

This syndrome is believed to be caused by a disorder of energy storage and utilization. However, this area is still undergoing intense medical research.

Signs and symptoms of metabolic syndrome

One of the major signs is central obesity that is also referred to as apple shaped adiposity. This is being overweight with accumulation of adipose tissue along the waist and torso of the body. Other signs are high blood pressure and insulin resistance among others.

Causes

The causes are still under research. The majority of sufferers are old, obese and have a level of resistance to insulin. Stress can also be a factor that contributes to this syndrome. Also, diet, genes, low physical activity and excessive use of alcohol are risk factors.

The current food environment also contributes to the development of this syndrome because it is not matched with our biochemistry. Gaining of weight is linked to this syndrome. The continuous provision of energy through carbohydrates, fats and protein and low physical activity creates a backlog of mitochondrion oxidation.

This process leads to dysfunction of the mitochondria and resistance of insulin. Furthermore, stress that is long term contributes to metabolic syndrome through disruption of the hormonal balance. This results in increased levels of glucose and insulin. This in return makes one more vulnerable to abdominal obesity as well as heart ailments and stroke. Moreover, central obesity is a common component of this syndrome. Being physically inactive is also associated with metabolic syndrome. People who are not active have more risks of developing this syndrome.

Several organizations have methods of diagnosing this syndrome. As per the national institutes of health guidelines, you suffer from metabolic syndrome if you have three or more of:

Large circumference of the waist - this is a waistline that measures at least thirty five inches in women and forty inches in men. This is also known as abdominal obesity or being apple shaped.

High level of triglyceride - if 150 mg dl or greater of this fat is found in your blood. Reduced high-density lipoprotein (HDL) cholesterol- this is cholesterol that is not harmful. It aids in the removal of cholesterol from the arteries. If it is less than 40 mg per deciliter in men and less than 50mg per deciliter in women.

Increased blood pressure - if it is 130/85 mmHg or higher. Blood pressure is the force of blood when it presses against your artery walls when the heart pumps. Elevated blood sugar-if it is 100mg/dl or higher.

The term metabolic means the biochemical processes that are involved in the normal functioning of the body.

Even though this syndrome was identified less than two decades ago, it is quite widespread. As per data from the American heart association, 47 million suffer from it. It runs in families and is more common in African American, Hispanics, Asians as well as Native Americans.

You may wonder why I touched on the metabolic syndrome.
Right? This is because the keto diet is a cure for all its symptoms.

Ketones
These are chemical structures of three ketone bodies: acetone, acetoacetic acid and beta- hydroxybutyric acid. They are produced by the liver from fatty acids during times that we have low food intake or when we fast. They are also produced when we have low carbs intake, starve or we intensely exercise.

The ketones are then picked up and converted so as to enter the citric acid cycle. From there, they are oxidized to release energy. Ketone bodies are produced through intense glucogenesis. This is the process of producing glucose from non-carb sources, but does not include fatty acids. Therefore, they are produced by the liver together with newly produced glucose after the liver's reserves have run out. They run out just within twenty four hours when fasting.

Also, ketone bodies have a unique scent which can be detected in the breath of people in ketosis and ketoacidosis. The scent is similar to the one for a nail polish remover. The ketone bodies are channeled into the bloodstream from the liver. The ketone bodies are then taken from the blood and converted into energy. The availability of high levels of ketone bodies in the bloodstream during starvation or during long periods of exercise and type 1 diabetes is called ketosis. In its extreme state, it is referred to as ketoacidosis.

Ketone bodies cannot be utilized by the liver for energy because it lacks the responsible enzymes. In normal people, ketone bodies are constantly produced by the liver and the concentration is maintained at around 1mg/dl. Their removal through urine is quite low and cannot be detected by using normal urine exams. When the rate of production of ketone bodies is more than their usage, their concentration increases in the blood stream. This is referred to as ketonemia. This is succeeded by ketonuria, which is the removal of ketone bodies through urine.

Ketonemia and ketonuria is referred to as ketosis. People who take diets that are low in carbs develop ketosis. This is at times referred to as nutritional ketosis. A blood test that is done in a laboratory is the most accurate and sure way of measuring ketones. It is recommended for people that suffer from diabetes whenever they feel ill. Symptoms such as nausea, vomiting or pain in the abdomen normally occur when the blood sugar is high. This may mean that you are suffering from diabetic ketoacidosis.

Home tests for ketone done on the blood or urine:
Monitors a person suffering from diabetes
Monitors a person on a diet with low carbs or high fats
Monitors a person who has difficulty in eating

How the test is done in a laboratory
A band that is elastic will be wrapped around the upper arm to stop blood flow. This enlarges the veins below the band and makes it easier to needle the vein.
The pierced area is cleaned using alcohol
The needle is inserted in the vein and more than one needle stick may be required

A tube is then attached to the needle so that it is filled with blood.
The band is then removed from the arm when enough blood is collected.
A gauze pad or cotton ball is applied over the pierced point as the needle is
removed. Pressure is then applied to the site and bandaged

Blood test at home

Some blood sugar meters can be used in measuring blood ketones. You use the
same method you use for measuring blood sugar.

If your blood sugar is at a normal range, and you are experiencing weight loss, the
presence of ketones may be perfectly normal.

However, if are diabetic, you need to watch your ketones and blood sugar. You
should test for ketones if:

- Your blood sugar is over 300
- The skin is flushed or changes color
- You vomit, have nausea or pains in the abdomen
- You feel lethargic
- You are thirstier than usual
- You have problems breathing
- Your breath smells fruity

Standard ketogenic diet - this refers to a very low-carb, moderate protein and high fat diet. Typically, it is composed of 75% fat, 20% protein and 5% carbs.

Cyclical ketogenic diet - this diet involves higher carb refeed periods, for instance 5 ketogenic days followed by 2 high carb days.

Targeted ketogenic diet - this diet enables you to add carbs during workouts High protein ketogenic diet-this is more or less the same as the standard keto diet, however, it is composed of more protein. The ratio is mostly 60% fat, 35% protein and 5% carbs.

However, you need to keep in mind that only the standard and high-protein ketogenic diets have been extensively studied. Additionally, the cyclical or targeted diets are more advanced methods that are primarily used by bodybuilders or athletes.

Healthy ketogenic diets

In case you feel like eating something between meals, the following are advised:

- Fatty fish or meat
- Cheese
- A handful of nuts
- Cheese with olives
- 1-2 hard-boiled eggs
- 90% dark chocolate

Great snacks for a ketogenic diet include pieces of meat, cheese, olives and dark chocolate.

Tips for eating out on a ketogenic diet
Several restaurants offer some kind of meat or fish, or dishes that are fish based. You can order this and replace foods containing high carbs with veggies. Meals that are egg based are also a good idea.

In short, when eating out, choose meat, fish or egg based foods. Also order extra vegetables rather than carbohydrates or starch.

Supplements for a ketogenic diet
Even though taking of supplements is not needed, some could prove helpful.

MCT oil - it is added to drinks or yogurt. It gives energy and aids in the increment of ketone levels.

Minerals - added salt and other minerals are useful when beginning the diet. This is because of the alterations in mineral and water balance.

Caffeine - can provide energy, aid in losing fat and enhance performance.

Exogenous ketones - this supplement can help in raising the levels of ketones in the body.

Creatine - this supplement has several benefits for one's health and performance. It is advisable if one combines ketogenic diets with exercise.
Whey- this increases the intake of daily protein.

Vegetarians and the keto diet

A vegetarian ketogenic diet would be regarded as the ultimate diet in terms of ethical consumption and fat loss. The traditional keto diet is based on the heavy consumption of animal fats; this is a contrast to the vegetarian diet.

A typical diet of a vegetarian is based on a high carbohydrate-to-fat macronutrient ratio, while the keto diet needs a high fat-to-carbohydrate macronutrient ratio.

You may be asking yourself if you could enjoy the benefits of ketosis while at the same time sticking to the vegetarian rules. Worry no more, the answer is yes.

The macronutrient ratio of the keto diet is not negotiable, therefore a high number of your calories have to originate from fat with very few soluble carbs. On the other hand, the consumption of animal products with veganism is also not negotiable.

Consequently, all meat and dairy products have to be avoided.

If you want to practice this diet, you need to know that it is so filling that you can shed weight without keeping track of calories or food. A study revealed that people on a keto diet lost 2.2 times more weight than those on a calorie-restricted low-fat diet. Furthermore, triglyceride and HDL cholesterol levels also improved. In a different study, it was also found out that people on the keto diet lost 3 times more weight than those on the diabetes UK's recommended diet. The fact is that a keto diet is more effective in weight loss as compared to a low-fat diet and it happens without hunger.

Losing weight by achieving optimal ketosis
The first and most important thing is to select a diet that is low in carbs.
Get into optimal ketosis. This is not recommended for sufferers of type 1 diabetics. The trick is to eat more fat. More fat in the food fills you more. This will make sure that you don't eat a lot of protein and carbohydrates. The insulin levels will go down and enable you reach optimal ketosis.

Being in optimal ketosis for a longer period of time will ensure that one experiences a maximum hormonal effect from eating a low carb diet. One can also order a ketone meter online and measure.

Ketosis, disease treatment and health
Far from burning fat, ketosis is beneficial for overall health and treatment of disease. Several cancers feed on glucose. Studies show that cancer has no ability to utilize ketones for the production of fuel, therefore they starve. The normal body cells have the metabolic flexibility to use ketone bodies for fuel. On the contrary, cancer does not.

Ketosis and improved focus as well as brain function

One of the causes of neurotoxicity is too much glucose. So, if the glucose supply is reduced, and the brain is prompted to burn ketones for fuel, a level occurs. Ketogenic diets also improve the functions of the brain through the process of clean fuel production.

Ketosis satiety

Your body should be in ketosis. The body should be able to utilize both ketones as well as glucose to produce fuel. As a sugar burner, the body has only one source to select from, and that is glucose. As a fat burner, it has two sources to select from. Furthermore, another benefit of fat burning is that it provides energy that is steady as well as long term. Also, when the body does not need sugar constantly, one achieves satiation and reduced hunger.

Ketosis is a state of the body being normal and healthy. It is a fact that many people undergo a phase of ketosis each morning after going without food while sleeping. This process also increases mitochondrial biogenesis. This is when new mitochondria are created inside our body cells. This results in an increase of more energy through efficient fuel production. Furthermore, ketosis increases the growth of more and more mitochondria. When mitochondria are few in the body, less energy is produced.

Ketosis also improves our functions of the brain because it has anti-oxidant effects. The body also has the ability to store carbs that can only last around two hours of exercise. After this, increased fatigue and decreased performance are experienced. The ketogenic diet is low on carbs and can help in optimizing the stores of stored glycogen found in the muscles.

Moreover, fat offers more energy at lower levels as compared to what carbs can provide in huge quantities.

In patients suffering from type 2 diabetes, this diet can be recommended. This is because with this type of diabetes, the body still produces some insulin but is not able to sufficiently use the insulin in the transportation of glucose into the cells to be used as fuel.

The ketogenic diet is focused on reducing intake of dietary carbohydrates. People suffering from type 2 diabetes are advised to reduce carbohydrate intake because they are converted to glucose and blood sugar levels are increased.

People suffering from diabetes who follow this diet need to carefully monitor their ketone levels.

The aim of ketogenic diet is the improvement of one's well-being through change in metabolism. You need to know:

- Who is not allowed to follow this diet
- How to begin this diet plan
- Worrying about the dangers of low carb diets
- Side effects of this diet
- Benefits of the ketogenic diet

Before starting a ketogenic diet plan, one should consult with a medical practitioner. This is mandatory for you to be informed of any pre- existing health conditions.

Basics

There are several ways by which one can implement a low carb ketogenic diet plan. But majority of them requires one to follow a higher fat, moderate protein and low carb food plan.one of the most popular ketogenic diets is the Atkins diet.

Several people believe that ketogenic diets are diets high in protein, but this is not true. Differences exist in how people relate low carb diet plans and ketogenic diet plans. These disparities revolve around the amount of carbohydrate and protein allowed on a day to day basis:

A ketogenic diet plan needs one to track the amount of carbs in the foods consumed and reduction of carbohydrate intake to an average of 40 grams in a day. For other people, consuming less than 100 grams in a day may be effective. However, this carb level is too high for the majority of people to achieve ketosis.

Additionally, the daily requirement for protein should be triggered by the aim or ideal body weight or lean body mass. Intake of protein also depends on height, gender and the amount of exercise that one does.

Too much of protein consumption can interfere with ketosis. The balance of calories after calculation of carbs and protein needs will be from fats. The ratios make sure that majority of people enter ketosis and remain in that state.

The nutrient intake on a ketogenic diet works out to about 70-75% of calories from fat, 20-25% from protein and 5-10% from carbohydrates every day when calories are not restricted. Even though counting of calories is not needed, it is vital to understand how the macronutrient percentages can be affected by consumption of calories.

The secret to implement a ketogenic diet in the correct manner is to keep in mind that you are alternating foods containing carbohydrates with more fats and moderate protein.

Fats have little effect, if any, on the levels of blood sugar as well as insulin. Protein affects both the levels of blood sugar and insulin.

If you consume a lot of protein for your ideal body weight, it can increase your levels of blood sugar and insulin will also be increased by protein temporarily.

Higher levels will affect the production of ketone bodies. Moreover, having a diet that has a lot of lean protein (with less fat) has the ability to make one sick.

How to start a ketogenic diet plan
One should understand the consequences of what will take place when intake of carbohydrate drops. You could follow the tips on the following page:

Get a carb counter guide

This will assist you in learning and recalling the amount of carbs in the foods that you eat. Counting of carbs is important in this diet plan and it is important for one to understand how it is done.

Go on a carbohydrate sweep

Inspect your food area and get rid of all foods that are high in carbs. This includes even whole grains.

Re stock the kitchen

Do this so that the foods that are low in carbohydrates are available. This will aid in keeping you on the right path. This diet is not a diet that needs special foods. You don't need to buy low carb packaged foodstuffs. Ketogenic foods are not highly processed foods. They are real whole foods that are close to their natural state. The only exception is the category of artificial sweeteners which are highly processed. Be ready to spend more time in the kitchen. This diet is all about cooking and eating foods that are real. If you don't know how to cook, learn now.

Give your meals thought and how you will plan them. This will aid you in buying the right foods from the grocery store.

Replace old habits with new ones.

Stay hydrated. As you lower carbohydrate intake, the kidneys will begin dumping excess water after being retained. Ensure that you take a lot of water to replace the one that is lost. If you find yourself experiencing headaches and muscle cramps, it means that you need more water. Stay clear of high carb foods because they will increase your levels of sugar and insulin. Additionally, cereal grains like wheat are toxic for most people.

Consider taking natural supplements.
You can also want to buy some testing kits so that you can find out if you are in ketosis. The reagent strip should not register as deep purple if you are using the ketones as a fuel source.

Keep a spreadsheet to track daily food intake and carb counts. Use one of the online food intake trackers or write it down in a journal. Far from keeping you on track, it will also aid you in recording the type of foods that you eat, how you feel and the changes that you make, so that if you are off track, you can refer.

Think of any social distractions and find ways of handling them.
You should also avoid focusing on your weight. Stop checking your weight on a daily basis. The body's weight varies on a daily basis because of differences in water intake and absorption. Furthermore, you will not have the ability to track loss of fat on a day to day basis. You can check your weight once in seven days.
Lastly, learn how to stop craving for sugar.

Is ketogenic diet safe?
The dangers of diets that are low in carbohydrates are just myths that people who have limited understanding of how this diet works say. The min fears are related to fat intake and the ketosis process.

Fears regarding fat
Majority of people are troubled by this diet plan because they are afraid of increasing the amount of fat that they consume.

This is true especially for saturated fats. For decades, people have been told how bad fat is. This message has been repeated over and over again, but it's not true.

A diet high in carbs raises blood sugar levels as well as insulin.

All that sugar and insulin is inflammatory. Even though saturated fat is healthy, it was blamed for causing heart ailments because it was studied together with a diet high in carbohydrates. A ketogenic diet that is high in saturated fats and very low in carbohydrate will reduce inflammation.

Saturated fats in the low carb diet context

According to a research from John Hopkins medical school, saturated fat has no harm in the context of a low carb diet. The ketogenic diet is healthier because the increased consumption of the saturated fat increases one's HDL cholesterol while at the same time, a diet low in carbs reduces the levels of triglycerides. These two factors are pointers when it comes to heart ailments.

The closer the triglyceride/HDL ratio is to 1, the healthier the heart. Heart disease is caused by high intake of carbohydrate rather than a high consumption of saturated fat and cholesterol.

The best way is to have a full blood test before you begin the ketogenic diet then follow the diet plan for ninety days. After that, do another blood test.

How people fare in ketosis

Even though evidence shows that a lot of people do well with reduced intake of carbohydrates, our bodies need at least 15 grams per day. This is because the ketogenic diet is a diet low on carbs but not zero carb diet. Do not get rid of carbohydrates completely.

General side effects of ketogenic diet

At first, switching to a ketogenic diet plan may be difficult because the metabolism of one's body is adapting to fat burning rather than depend on glucose. However, it's good to know that most of the symptoms can be avoided.

During the first seven days on this diet, the levels of blood sugar will drop and one may experience an overload of insulin and reactive hypothermia. This usually happens to people who are resistant to insulin.

It takes approximately three days to burn through all the glycogen that is stored in the muscles and liver. A ketogenic diet also has the ability to alter the water and mineral balance of a person's body, so, adding extra salt to the food and taking mineral supplements may be helpful. Try taking sodium, potassium and magnesium on a daily basis to reduce the side effects.

Benefits and dangers

If you follow a ketogenic diet plan, and adapted to it, you will feel much better and healthier. One of the health gains of this diet is that it will lower your fasting blood sugar as well as the levels of insulin. Furthermore, it also aids in the reversal of insulin resistant conditions such as type 2 diabetes, fatty liver and metabolic syndrome.

In case you have doubts, please remember that there is a lot of credible research that has shown how following a ketogenic diet plan is not harmful to the health of humans.it is only when one consumes too much fat and a lot of carbs that you negatively impact on your health.

The sugar that comes from the carbohydrates increases the levels of insulin and those high levels of insulin interrupt the normal fat metabolism. More fat is stored or circulated in the blood stream.

This results in the metabolic syndrome and weight that is linked with resistance of insulin and begins the health issues associated with a diet high in carbohydrates, not a ketogenic diet plan.

This diet aids in losing weight

A ketogenic diet is an effective way of losing weight apart from lowering risks of ailments. Research has revealed that ketogenic diets are far more effective than the recommended low fat diets. Furthermore, the ketogenic diet is so filling that one can shed weight without counting calories or monitoring the food you eat.

Another study also found out that people on a ketogenic diet lost two times more weight than those on a calorie restricted low fat diet plan. Their triglyceride as well as HDL levels also improved. It was also found out in a separate study that people on a ketogenic diet lost three times more weight than those on the diabetes recommended diet.

Several reasons exist as to why a ketogenic diet is better than a low fat diet.one of them is the increased consumption of protein which offers benefits. In a nutshell, ketogenic diets aid one in losing weight than diets with low fat. All this happens without hunger.

Ketogenic diet for diabetes and prediabetes

This diet enables you to lose excessive fat, which is closely connected to type 2 diabetes, prediabetes as well as metabolic syndrome.

Several studies have been done to prove that this diet aids with diabetes. One of them found out that this diet improved the sensitivity of insulin by a whopping 75%.

Another also investigated people with type 2 diabetes. It found out that seven out of the twenty one participants were able to stop all medications related to diabetes. All these show that this diet has the ability to boost insulin sensitivity and trigger loss of fat, which results in the improvement of type 2 diabetes and prediabetes.

Other health benefits

The ketogenic diet originally came about as a tool for the treatment of neurological disorders like epilepsy. It also has the ability to improve body fat, HDL levels, blood pressure and blood sugar. Furthermore, this diet is also being used in the treatment of several cancer types and slowing of tumor growths. It also reduces the symptoms of Alzheimer's and slows down its progress. In epilepsy, it reduces seizures. It improves the symptoms of Parkinson's.

Since this diet reduces the levels of insulin, it plays a key role in polycystic ovary syndrome.

A study also found out that the ketogenic diet reduces concussions and aids in recovery for those with brain injuries.

For those suffering from acne, lower levels of insulin as well as consumption of less sugar and processed foods is beneficial.

They suppress appetite in a good way

Feeling hungry is the worst side effect of being on a diet. It is one of the major reasons that many people give up on their dieting programs. One of the advantages of eating a low carb diet leads to an automatic appetite reduction. Studies have shown that when people cut carbs and consume more protein and fat, they end up consuming fewer calories.

A lot of fat loss happens in the abdominal cavity

Not all fats in the body are alike. Where fat is stored determines how it affects health as well as the risk of illness.it is important to know that we have fat under the skin and in the abdominal cavity. The fat that tends to be lodged around the organs is what is known as visceral fat. A lot of fat in such areas can trigger inflammation, resistance to insulin and is responsible for metabolism syndrome. Diets that are low in carbs are quite effective in the reduction of such abdominal fat that is harmful.

Reduction of triglycerides

Triglycerides are molecules of fat. Consumption of carbs drives up levels of triglycerides, especially sugar. When a person cuts down on carbs, they experience a reduction in blood triglycerides.

Increased levels of good cholesterol

The higher the levels of HDL, the lower the risk of heart ailments. One of the best ways to raise levels of HDL is to consume fat and diets low in carb.

Reduction of blood sugar and insulin levels

When we consume carbohydrates, they are broken down into glucose in the digestive tract. Thereafter, they enter the bloodstream and raise the levels of blood sugar. Since high levels of blood sugar is toxic, the body responds through insulin.

For healthy people, the rapid response of insulin minimizes the blood sugar surge in order to prevent it from being harmful to us.

However, many people have resistance of insulin. This means that the cells do not detect the insulin making it difficult for the body to take blood sugar into the cells.

This can lead to type 2 diabetes.by reducing intake of carbs, you eliminate the need for insulin. Both the blood sugar and insulin levels decrease.

Reduction of blood pressure

Low carb diets are effective in the reduction of blood pressure and this reduces the risk of diseases.

Ketogenic diet is the most effective in the treatment of metabolic syndrome
The symptoms are:

- Abdominal obesity
- Increased blood pressure
- Increased fasting blood sugar levels
- High triglycerides
- Low HDL levels

All these symptoms improve on a low carb diet.

They improve the pattern of LDL cholesterol
This is bad cholesterol and is linked to heart attacks. A diet that is low on carbs transform LDL particles from small to large, and at the same time reducing the number of LDL particles that float in the bloodstream.

Several versions of the ketogenic exist:

Standard ketogenic diet - this is a very low carb, moderate protein and high fat diet. It consists of 75% fat, 20% protein and 5% carbohydrates.

Cyclical ketogenic diet - this diet is about periods of higher carb refeeds such as five ketogenic days succeeded by two days of high carb.

Targeted ketogenic diet - this diet allows one to add carbohydrates when working out

High protein ketogenic diet - this is the same as the standard ketogenic diet but it contains more protein. The ratio is 60% fat, 35% protein and 5% carbohydrates.

It is important to note that only the standard and high protein ketogenic diets have been studied thoroughly. Cyclical and targeted ketogenic diets are methods that are more advanced and primarily used by athletes or body builders. Of all these diets, the standard ketogenic diet is the most known and recommended.

Keto macros

Macro refers to macronutrients. Your macros are the daily intake of the three major nutrients; they are fats, protein and carbs. You are advised to maintain your carb intake less than 30g per day and protein between 0.7g- 1.2g per pound of lean body mass.

Keto flu

Even though ketosis is usually safe, it is common to experience some side effects that clear with time. People transitioning from sugar-burning to fat-burning will undergo side effects. This condition is known as the keto flu because the symptoms are similar to those of flu; nausea, headache, and cramps. You are advised to drink water with salt and lemon. Additionally, you will need to gradually reduce your carb intake. When starting on the keto diet, you lose water and electrolytes. This occurs because carbs retain water and salts in the body. So, when you stop carb intake, your body loses water.

In case the keto flu is due to too little hydration, drinking a glass of salty water with lemon can help. When you exclude carbs from your diet, the brain will slightly run low on energy before it adapts to using ketone bodies to generate fuel instead of sugar.

Carbohydrate metabolism

This is the process that involves forming, breaking down and conversion of carbs in living things. The most common carbohydrate is glucose. The normal cells of the body metabolize food nutrients and oxygen during cellular respiration. A huge portion of this energy production takes place in the mitochondria.

Any foods that are high in carbohydrates should be limited. One should cut down on sugary foods, grains or starches, fruits, beans, root veggies and tubers, low fat diets, selected sauces, booze and sugar free diets.

French fries and potato chips
They contain a lot of calories and one can consume a lot of them. Consumption of fries and potato chips is connected to gaining of weight. A study revealed that these foods contribute to gaining of weight than any other food. Furthermore, baked, roasted or froes potatoes contain cancer causing ingredients. It is advisable to eat plain, boiled potatoes. French fries and potato chips are fattening and unhealthy.

Drinks that are sugary
Beverages like soda are one of the unhealthiest foods on earth. They are strongly linked to gaining of weight and are detrimental to one's health if taken in excess. Liquid calories do not make you feel satisfied and you will add these calories on top of your normal intake. If you want to lose weight, steer clear of these drinks.

White bread
It is highly refined and contains lots of added sugars. It ranks high on the glycemic index and can raise levels of sugar. A study revealed that eating two slices of white bread in a day was linked to a greater risk of adding weight and being obese. Bread that is made from very fine flour can raise sugar levels and cause one to overeat.

Candy bars
They are quite unhealthy because they stack a lot of sugar, added oils and refined flour. Furthermore, they are high in calories and low in nutritive value. An average candy bar contains an average of 250 calories. If you crave for snacks, eat a fruit or nuts.

Most fruit juices

Many of the fruit juices found in stores have very little similarity to the whole fruit. They are highly processed and contain a lot of sugar. They contain as much sugar as soda or even more. These juices also contain no fibers and they will not have the same effect as real fruits.

Pastries and cakes

They have unhealthy ingredients such as added sugar and refined flour. Furthermore, they also contain artificial Trans- fats which are very harmful and connected to several diseases. Additionally, they are less satisfying and you will feel hungry very fast after eating them.

Alcohol

It provides more calories than carbohydrates and protein. Consumption of alcohol in moderation is okay; however, heavy drinking is linked to increased gaining of weight. Beer causes gaining of weight.

Ice cream

This is quite unhealthy, high in calories and loaded with sugar. Think about making your own ice cream using less sugar and healthier ingredients like yogurt and fruit. Additionally, serve yourself small portions so as to avoid eating too much.

Pizza

Ones that are made commercially are very unhealthy. They contain high calories and often contain unhealthy ingredients such as refined flour and meat that is processed. It is better to make pizzas at home because they are healthier.

Coffee drinks with high calories

They are loaded with empty calories that can be the same as a whole meal. Plain, black coffee is very healthy and can aid in fat burning. However, such drinks have artificial ingredients that are very unhealthy and fattening.

Foods with a lot of added sugar
Examples are sugary breakfast cereals and flavored yogurt.

Soy sauce
Even though it is low on calories, it has high sodium content that can make you bloated and increase your chances of getting hypertension.

Tropical fruits
There are some to avoid if you want to lose weight. Take limited mangoes and ripe pineapples because they contain a lot of sugar.
Foods to eat

You should consume plenty of meat, fatty fish, eggs, butter and cream, cheese, nuts and seeds, healthy oils, avocados, low carb veggies and condiments.
A sample ketogenic meal plan for fourteen days:

Day one
    Breakfast: bacon, eggs and tomatoes
    Lunch: chicken salad, olive oil and feta cheese
    Supper: salmon and asparagus cooked in butter

Day two
    Breakfast: egg, tomato, basil and goat cheese omelet
    Lunch: almond milk, peanut butter, cocoa powder and stevia milkshake
    Supper: meatballs, cheddar cheese and veggies

Day three
    Breakfast: ketogenic milkshake
    Lunch: salad made from shrimp, olive oil and avocado
    Supper: pork chops, parmesan cheese, broccoli and salad

Day four

     Breakfast: omelet, avocado, salsa, peppers, onion and spice

     Lunch: nuts, celery sticks, guacamole and salsa

     Supper: chicken stuffed with pesto and cream cheese and veggies

Day five

     Breakfast: yogurt that is sugar free, peanut butter, cocoa powder and stevia

     Lunch: stir fry cooked beef in coconut oil and veggies

     Supper: bun-less burger, bacon, egg and cheese

Day six

     Breakfast: ham and cheese omelet, veggies

     Lunch: ham and cheese slices, nuts

     Supper: white fish, egg, spinach cooked in coconut oil

Day seven

     Breakfast: fried eggs, bacon and mushrooms

     Lunch: burger with salsa, cheese and guacamole

     Supper: steak, eggs and side salad

Day eight

     Breakfast: vanilla keto smoothie

     Lunch: easy avocado and egg salad. Rather than using sour cream, use mayo

     Supper: pork chops with keto gravy served with creamy keto mash

Day nine

     Breakfast: pumpkin pie chia pudding

     Lunch: salmon stuffed avocado

     Supper: perfect ribeye steak with gremolata served with creamy keto mash

Day ten

    Breakfast: pesto scrambled eggs

    Lunch: classic tricolore salad

    Dinner: pan-roasted salmon with creamy keto mash

Day eleven

    Breakfast: chocolate keto smoothie

    Lunch: easy avocado and egg salad

    Supper: spicy chorizo meatballs served with buttered Brussels sprouts

Day twelve

    Breakfast: pesto scrambled eggs

    Lunch: classic tricolore salad

    Supper: spicy chorizo meatballs served with buttered Brussels sprouts

Day thirteen

    Breakfast: zucchini breakfast hash

    Lunch: healthy mackerel salad

    Supper: spicy chorizo meatballs

Day fourteen

    Breakfast: All day keto breakfast

    Lunch: salmon stuffed avocado

    Supper: spicy chorizo meatballs

Always try and alternate the veggies and meat over time since each type gives different nutrients and health benefits.

Commonly asked questions about the ketogenic diet

Is one allowed to eat carbohydrates again?
Yes, one can, even though it is advisable to get rid of them when starting. After sixty to ninety days, one can eat carbs once in a while.

Does one lose muscles?
In any diet, the risks of losing muscles exist. However, with ketogenic diet, you reduce the chances of muscle loss, especially if you lift weights.

Can this diet aid in building muscle?
Yes it can. However, it may not be effective like on a moderate carb diet plan.

Does one need to refeed or load carbs?
Nope, although a few days with high calorie foods may be beneficial

How much protein is one required to eat?
The quantity of protein has to be moderate because very high amounts can raise the levels of insulin and lower ketones. A maximum of 35% of the total calorie intake is recommended.

How to deal with fatigue?
Lower the intake of carbs and refer to the above tips.

Why does urine and breath smell?
Urine smell is due to removal of byproducts created during ketosis. For fresh breath, chew some sugar free gum or drink naturally flavored water.

Several ways of losing weight exist, but others can be harmful to one's health. This book provides you with all you need to know about the ketogenic diet. This diet plan can be practiced by people of all ages, both the young and old. This diet often scares people because many think that you will have to give up all the good foods you enjoy. However, this is not true. There are still healthy snacks and main meals that one can have on this diet. Another thing that scares people is the initial hunger as well as the side effects felt when starting this diet.

However, these side effects don't stick for long because the body adapts so fast. This diet increases our mental as well as physical performance because of the energy produced while on this diet.

It is good to consult your doctor before starting this diet especially if you have underlying medical conditions.

While on this diet, a person should consume lots of healthy protein and fats and cut down on carbohydrates. Please not that you don't have to completely eliminate carbs from your diet. You just keep it at a low.

Keto egg beef - Ingredients for two portions

Ingredients

- Extra lean ground beef
- Eight egg whites
- Two cups of baby spinach,
  (can also use regular spinach)
- Tomatoes, either four small ones
  or two Italian ones
- Half cup of red peppers
- Sea salt and black pepper to taste

Nutritional value per serving
Calories are 250
Protein is 50 grams
Carbohydrates is 6 grams
Fat is 2 grams

Since you are on a ketogenic diet, you will need higher amounts of fat. You are advised to keep the yolks, avoid using extra lean meat, and add olive or coconut oil to the recipe. You can also add bacon. This should take around five minutes to prepare and ten minutes to cook.

How to prepare

1. Pre heat a medium pan that is non- sticky to medium heat. You can add olive oil to ensure that it doesn't stick.
2. Add the beef to the hot skillet and break it into large pieces.
3. Break the beef into smaller pieces until it is fully cooked. You then put it in a bowl that is set aside.
4. Scramble the egg whites until they are dry and put them over the meat
5. Lightly sauté the tomatoes, spinach, red peppers and basil
6. Put the veggies over the meat and eggs and serve

This is easy to make. According to a scientific study conducted in Zurich, the vitamin B3, also known as niacin, which is found in bacon, has the ability to prolong one's lifespan. If you want scrambled eggs that are light and fluffy, the secret is to move them constantly to avoid them taking on any color. One can also add milk or heavy milk if he wishes.

Ingredients

Eggs

- Three large eggs
- One tablespoon of unsalted butter
- Coarse salt and pepper that is freshly ground

Bacon

<table>
<tr><td>

Nutritional value

Calories are 318

Fat is 26.3 grams

Carbohydrates is 1.8 grams

Protein is 17.4 grams

Calories are 200

Fats are 19 grams

Carbohydrates is zero

Protein is 7 grams

</td></tr>
</table>

How to prepare

1. Beat the eggs together using a fork
2. Using low heat, melt the butter in a medium non-stick skillet
3. Add the egg mixture
4. Using a heatproof flexible spatula, pull eggs to the center of the pan gently and let the liquid parts run out under the perimeter. Cook, while moving the eggs continually using the spatula until the eggs are set. This takes an average of two and a half minutes
5. Season it with salt and pepper, serve while still hot

In a skillet

Many people prefer the cast iron skillet; however, any kind of skillet can work. One may also require a set of tongs to aid in the grasping of the hot slices as well as flipping them. Because bacon cooks best when you go low and slow, set the skillet over heat that is medium.

As soon as the pan has heated, lay down the bacon in a single layer and let the strips cook for a few minutes without movement. The pan is not usually oiled at first because the bacon releases so much grease so fast. As soon as they begin curling up, flip the slices over to the other side and cook until they become crispy to your preference. Place the cooked slices on a paper tissue so as to drain as you cook the remaining pieces. Pour off the bacon fat in batches to avoid your slices being greasy.

In the Oven

This is recommended when cooking a lot of bacon at a time, especially because it leaves the stove free for other cooking. Pre heat the oven to 350 degrees and put the bacon on a baking sheet lined with paper foil. Bake it for an average of twenty minutes and then place the bacon on paper tissues to drain oil and firm it up.

In the microwave

This is the preferred option if one is in a hurry. Just line the microwave plate with a few sheets of paper towels and arrange the bacon in one layer. Put the microwave on high for five minutes on average until the bacon is cooked the way you like it.

This is a quick, delicious and clean recipe for losing weight.one can use chocolate protein powder to add some protein and offer it a delicious milk chocolate taste, but you can instead use cocoa powder. Chia seeds are one of the best foods that aid in faster burning of fats. This is because they are loaded with fiber, omega 3, antioxidants as well as minerals. Furthermore, they expand in the stomach to keep one full and reduce appetite. They are also gluten free because they are seeds and not grains.

Ingredients

- Three tablespoons of chia seeds
- One cup of unsweetened almond milk.
  (However, you can use skim milk
  or soya milk instead.)
- A quarter cup of fresh or frozen raspberries
- One scoop of protein powder.
  (This can be alternated with cocoa powder,
  you can also use a teaspoon of honey if
  you wish even though it is not important
  if you use protein powder.)

Nutritional value per serving
Calories are 235
Protein is 30 grams
Carbs are 19 grams
Fat is 12 grams
Fiber is 8 grams

How to prepare

1. Mix the almond milk and the chocolate protein powder. Use a fork to stir well
2. Add the chia seeds and mix well using a fork
3. Leave the mix for five minutes then stir
4. Stir it again after five minutes and let it rest for half an hour in the fridge
5. Serve and add the raspberries on top

Mustard seed - boosts metabolism even after 24 hours after consuming it
Black pepper - aids in faster digestion
Ginger - hinders absorption of cholesterol
Cinnamon - aids in better carb processing
Cayenne pepper - burns fat

Ketogenic white pizza frittata (for 8 servings)

These are great when microwaved, re heated in the oven or just plain cold. This recipe makes use of different cheeses in the frittata base and a top with mozzarella and pepperoni combo. Inside you find spinach that makes sure we get some greens. The texture is a bit more on the dense side for a frittata due to the melted ricotta and parmesan cheese inside.

Ingredients

- Twelve large eggs
- 9 oz. bag of frozen spinach
- 1 oz. pepperoni
- 5 oz. mozzarella cheese
- One teaspoon of minced garlic
- Half a cup of fresh ricotta cheese
- Half a cup of parmesan cheese
- Four tablespoons of olive oil
- A quarter teaspoon of nutmeg
- Salt and pepper

Nutrient intake per serving
Calories are 298
Carbs are 2.1g
Fat is 23.8g
Protein is 19.4g

How to prepare

1. Place the frozen spinach into the microwave for between 3-4 minutes or until defrosted. However, it should not be hot. Squeeze the spinach using your hands and drain as much water as you can. Set it aside.
2. Pre heat the oven to 375F. Mix the eggs, olive oil and spices. Whisk well until properly mixed.
3. Add in the ricotta cheese, parmesan cheese and spinach. Break the spinach into small pieces using your hands while adding.
4. Pour the mixture into a cast iron skillet then sprinkle mozzarella cheese on the top. Add pepperoni on top of that.
5. Bake it for half an hour. In case you are using a glass container in place of cast iron, bake it for 45 minutes or until it is completely set.
6. Slice it up and devour it. You can top it up using crème fraiche, ranch dressing or your favorite fatty sauce.

These breakfast muffins are rich, hearty and moist. Far from that, they are low in carbs and high in fibers because of their flaxseed base and wholesome ingredients. Each muffin offers a rich and dark taste of chocolate with a hint of caramel. These muffins are satisfying and can keep you full until lunch hour. Furthermore, they are not hard to make.

Ingredients

- A cup of golden flaxseed meal
- A quarter cup of cocoa powder
- A tablespoon of cinnamon
- Half a tablespoon of baking powder
- Half a teaspoon of salt
- A large egg
- Two tablespoons of coconut oil
- A quarter cup of sugar
  free caramel syrup
- Half a cup of pumpkin puree
- A teaspoon of vanilla extract
- A teaspoon of apple cider vinegar
- A quarter cup of silvered almonds

Nutrient intake per serving
Calories are 183
Carbs are 3.3g
Fat is 13.4g
Protein is 7g

How to prepare

1. Pre heat the oven to 350F and mix all the dry ingredients in a mixing bowl
2. In a different bowl, mix all the wet ingredients
3. You then pour all the wet ingredients into the dry ingredients and mix well
4. Line a muffin tin with paper liners and spoon about a quarter cup of batter into each liner. Sprinkle the silvered almonds over each muffin and gently press for them to stick. Bake in the oven for a quarter of an hour.
5. Enjoy when warm or cool

They take less time to make and store. They contain 1.5g net carbs per muffin. When fresh, their bottoms crust up well and add the extra crunch when they come out of the oven.

Ingredients

- Three quarters of a cup of blanched almond flour
- A quarter cup of golden flaxseed meal
- A third of a cup of erythritol
- A tablespoon of baking powder
- Two tablespoons of poppy seeds
- A quarter cup of salted butter that is melted
- A quarter cup of heavy cream
- Three large eggs
- Zest of two lemons
- Three tablespoons of lemon juice
- A tablespoon of vanilla extract
- Twenty five drops of liquid stevia

Nutrient intake per serving
Calories are 129
Carbs are 1.5g
Fat is 11.3g
Protein is 3.7g

How to prepare

1. Pre heat the oven to 350F. In a bowl, use a fork to mix the almond flour, flaxseed meal, erythritol and poppy seeds.
2. Stir in the melted butter, eggs and the heavy cream until smooth. Make sure that there are no lumps in the batter
3. Once it becomes smooth, add in the baking powder, liquid stevia, vanilla extract, lemon zest and lemon juice. Mix thoroughly
4. Divide the batter equally among 12 cupcake molds.
5. Bake for twenty minutes or until they slightly turn brown.
6. Remove from the oven and let it cool for ten minutes

The bacon offers a burst of flavor with the eggs and cheese. The chives offer a sweet onion taste.

Ingredients

- Two slices of cooked bacon
- A teaspoon of bacon fat
- Two large eggs
- 1 oz. of cheddar cheese
- Two stalks chives
- Salt and pepper

Nutrient intake per serving
Calories are 463
Carbs are 1g
Fat is 39g
Protein is 24g

How to prepare

1. Ensure that you have all the ingredients ready because the omelet cooks quite fast. Shred the cheese, precook the bacon and chop the chives
2. Heat a pan with bacon fat in it at a medium low heat. Add the eggs then season with chives, salt and pepper.
3. As soon as the edges start to set, add the bacon to the center and let it cook for around thirty seconds longer. You then turn off the heat
4. Add the cheese on top the bacon and make sure it's centered. You then take two edges of the omelet and fold them onto the cheese. Hold the edges for a moment as the cheese partially melts to act as an adhesive to hold them in place.
5. Do the same with the other edges creating a burrito of sorts. You then flip it over and let it cook for a little longer in the warm pan
6. Serve with extra cheese, bacon and chives if you like.

This is an option for a brunch or heavy breakfast.

Ingredients

- 4 oz. sausage
- 2 oz. pepper jack cheese
- 4 slices of bacon
- 2 large eggs
- A tablespoon of butter
- A tablespoon of PB fit powder
- Salt and pepper

<table>
<tr><td>Nutrient intake per serving</td></tr>
<tr><td>Carbs are 3g</td></tr>
<tr><td>Fat is 56g</td></tr>
<tr><td>Protein is 30.5g</td></tr>
<tr><td>Calories are 655</td></tr>
</table>

How to prepare

1. Begin by cooking the bacon. Lay the strips on a wire rack over a cookie sheet. Bake at 400F for 25 minutes or until crisp.
2. Mix together butter and PB fit powder in a small container to rehydrate. Set aside
3. Form sausage patties and cook in a pan over medium to high heat. Turn over when the bottom side is browned
4. Grate the cheese and have it ready
5. As soon as the other side of the sausage patty is browned, add the cheese and cover with a lid
6. Remove the sausage patties with the melted cheese and set aside. Fry an egg in the same pan
7. Bring everything together; sausage patty, egg, bacon and the rehydrated PB fit on top.

This takes about 10 minutes to prepare.

Ingredients

- Six hot dogs
- 12 slices of bacon
- 2 oz. cheddar cheese
- Half a teaspoon of garlic powder
- Half a teaspoon of onion powder
- Salt and pepper

<table>
<tr><td>Nutrient intake per serving</td></tr>
<tr><td>Carbs are 0.3g</td></tr>
<tr><td>Fat is 34.5g</td></tr>
<tr><td>Protein is 16.8g</td></tr>
<tr><td>Calories are 380</td></tr>
</table>

How to prepare

1. Heat the oven to 400F. Slit all the hotdogs to create space for cheese.
2. Slice 2 oz. cheddar cheese into small and long rectangles.
3. Stuff them into the hotdogs.
4. Tightly wrap one slice of bacon around the hotdog
5. Go on and tightly wrap a second slice of bacon around the hotdog. Make sure it slightly overlaps with the first slice.
6. Poke each side of the bacon and hotdog with a toothpick, so as to secure the bacon in place.
7. You then set on a wire rack that's on top of a cookie sheet. Season with garlic powder, onion powder, salt and pepper.
8. Bake for between 35-40 minutes or until the bacon becomes crispy. You can also broil the bacon on top if needed.
9. Serve with some nice creamed spinach

Their crispy outside combines with the soft creamy filling on the inside.

Ingredients

- 10 oz. canned and drained tuna
- A quarter cup of mayonnaise
- A cubed medium avocado
- A quarter cup of parmesan cheese
- A third of a cup of almond flour
- Half a teaspoon of garlic powder
- A quarter teaspoon of onion powder
- Salt and pepper
- Half a cup of coconut oil for frying

Nutrient intake per serving
Carbs are 0.8g
Fat is 11.8g
Protein is 6.2g
Calories are 135

How to prepare

1. Drain a can of tuna and add to a large sized container where everything will be mixed
2. Add mayonnaise, parmesan cheese and spices to the tuna and mix well
3. Slice the avocado into half and cube it
4. Add avocado into the tuna mixture and fold together. Try not to mash the avocado into the mixture
5. Form the tuna mixture into balls and roll into almond flour, covering them completely. Set aside
6. Heat the coconut oil in a pan over medium heat. As soon as it's hot, add the tuna balls and fry until all sides are crisp
7. Remove from the pan and serve

Ingredients

Keto cloud bread

- 3 large eggs
- 3 oz. cream cheese
- An eighth of a teaspoon cream of tartar
- A quarter teaspoon of salt
- Half a teaspoon of garlic powder

Filling

- A tablespoon of mayonnaise
- A teaspoon of sriracha
- Two bacon slices
- 3 oz. chicken
- Two pepper jack cheese slices
- 2 grape tomatoes
- A quarter medium avocado

<u>Nutrient intake per serving</u>
Carbs are 2g
Fat is 28.3g
Protein is 22g
Calories are 361

How to prepare

1. Preheat the oven to 300F. Start by separating 3 eggs into two clean dry bowls.
2. Add the cream of tartar and salt to the egg whites. Use an electric mixer to whip the whites until they become soft and foamy.
3. In a separate bowl, mix 3 oz. of cubed cream cheese with the egg yolks and beat until they become pale yellow
4. Gently fold the egg whites into the yolks, half at a time
5. On a parchment paper lined baking sheet, spoon a quarter cup of the keto cloud bread batter.
6. Use a spatula to gently press the tops of the keto cloud bread to form squares. You then sprinkle the tops with garlic powder and bake for about 25 minutes
7. As the keto cloud bread is baking, cook the chicken and bacon with salt and pepper
8. You arrange the sandwich by combining mayo and sriracha and spreading it on the underside of one keto cloud bread. Add the chicken into the mayo mixture.
9. Add the two slices of pepper jack cheese and the bacon. Nestle some halved grape tomatoes and spread the mashed avocado on top. Season to taste and top with the other keto cloud bread.

Tofu that is baked is quite delicious. You get a rich cube that is full of flavor and crunchy on the outsides. Furthermore, raw bok choy is fantastic. It is crunchy and offers a distinct taste to the salad.

Ingredients

Oven baked tofu

- 15 oz. extra firm tofu
- A tablespoon of soy sauce
- A tablespoon of sesame oil
- A tablespoon of water
- Two teaspoons of minced garlic
- A tablespoon of rice wine vinegar
- Juice made from half a lemon

Bok choy salad

- 9 oz. bok choy
- A stalk of green onion
- Two tablespoons of chopped cilantro
- Three tablespoons of coconut oil
- Two tablespoons of soy sauce
- A tablespoon of sambal olek
- A tablespoon of peanut butter
- Juice from half a lime
- Seven drops of liquid stevia

Nutrient intake per serving
Carbs are 5.7g
Fat is 35g
Protein is 25g
Calories are 442

1. Begin by pressing the tofu. Place the tofu in a kitchen towel and put something heavy over it. It takes about 4-6 hours to dry out. However, you may need to change the kitchen towel when half way done.
2. After pressing the tofu, work on the marinade. Mix all the ingredients for the marinade; that is soy sauce, sesame oil, water, garlic, vinegar and lemon
3. Chop the tofu into squares and place them in a plastic bag together with the marinade. Let it marinate for at least half an hour. However, overnight is preferred
4. Pre heat the oven to 350F. Place the tofu on a baking sheet lined with parchment paper. Bake for half an hour.
5. When the tofu is cooked, start on the bok choy salad. Chop the cilantro and spring onion
6. You then mix all the other ingredients together apart from lime juice and bok choy. You then add cilantro and the spring onion. You can also microwave the coconut oil for about ten seconds so that it melts
7. When the tofu is almost cooked, add the lime juice into the salad dressing and mix together.
8. Chop the bok choy into small pieces
9. Remove the tofu from the oven and assemble the salad with tofu, bok choy and sauce

In the ketogenic diet, fatty fish has proven that it lowers levels of cholesterol and aid with the overall health. This recipe is easy to prepare and super tasty. It takes under 15 minutes to prepare.

Ingredients

- Half a cup of walnuts
- Two tablespoons of sugar free maple syrup
- Half a tablespoon of Dijon mustard
- A quarter teaspoon of dill
- Two, 3 oz. salmon fillets
- A tablespoon of olive oil
- Salt and pepper

Nutrient intake per serving
Carbs are 3g
Fat is 43g
Protein is 20g
Calories are 373

How to prepare

1. Preheat the oven to 350F. add half a cup of walnuts to the food processor
2. Add two tablespoons of maple syrup and the spices
3. Add a tablespoon of mustard
4. Pulse this in the food processor until it is paste like
5. Heat a pan or skillet with a tablespoon of oil until very hot. Thoroughly dry the salmon fillets and place them skin down in the pan. Let it sear for about 3 minutes, undisturbed.
6. As it sears, add the walnut mixture to the top side of the salmon fillets
7. After that, transfer them to an oven and bake for about 8 minutes
8. Serve with fresh spinach and enjoy.
9. You can sprinkle with a little bit of smoked paprika

Ingredients

<table>
<tr><td>

- A teaspoon of coriander seeds
- Two tablespoons of olive oil
- Two sliced chili peppers
- Two cups of chicken broth
- Two cups of water
- A teaspoon of turmeric
- Half a teaspoon of ground cumin
- Four tablespoons of tomato paste
- 16 oz. chicken thighs
- Two tablespoons of butter
- A medium avocado
- 2 oz. queso fresco
- Four tablespoons of fresh chopped cilantro
- Juice from half a lime
- Salt and pepper

</td><td>

<u>Nutrient intake per serving</u>
Carbs are 5.8g
Fat is 27.8g
Protein is 28g
Calories are 396

</td></tr>
</table>

How to prepare

1. Cut and set the chicken thighs to cook in an oiled pan. Season it with salt and pepper. You then leave it aside to rest.
2. In two tablespoons of olive oil, heat up the coriander seeds to release more flavor
3. Once they are fragrant, add in the sliced chili peppers to add their flavor to the oil
4. You then add in the broth and water.
5. Let it simmer and season.
6. Add turmeric, ground cumin, salt and pepper to taste
7. As the soup simmers, add in the tomato paste and butter. Stir so that it melts and mixes.
8. Let the soup simmer for between 5-10 minutes.
9. Lower the heat on the stove and the juice from half the lime
10. Place four ounces of chicken thighs into the bottom of the bowl so that you are able to pour soup over it.
11. Ladle the soup for serving. Garnish with a quarter of an avocado into each bowl, half an ounce of queso fresco and cilantro

Ingredients

- One ½ lbs. chicken thighs, bone-in-skin-on
- 1 lb. chicken thighs, boneless, skinless
- Two tablespoons of olive oil
- Two teaspoons of onion powder
- Three cloves of minced garlic
- An inch of grated ginger root
- Three tablespoons of tomato paste
- Five teaspoons of garam masala
- Two teaspoons of smoked paprika
- Four teaspoons of kosher salt
- 10oz can of diced tomatoes
- A cup of heavy cream & cup coconut milk
- Fresh chopped cilantro
- A teaspoon of guar gum

Nutrient intake per serving
Carbs are 5.8g
Fat is 41.2g
Protein is 26g
Calories are 493

How to prepare

1. De bone the chicken on the bone-in chicken thighs. Chop all the chicken pieces into bite sized pieces. Ensure that you keep the skin for the pieces that have it.
2. Add the chicken to a slow cooker and grate an inch of ginger over the top
3. Add all the dry spices into the slow cooker and mix properly
4. Add canned diced tomatoes and tomato paste into the slow cooker and mix well once more
5. Finally, add half a cup of coconut milk and mix well. Cook over low heat for 6 hours or 3 hours over high heat.
6. Once the slow cooker is over, add the remainder of the coconut milk, heavy cream and guar gum and mix well into the chicken. This will help the curry thicken nicely.
7. Serve over cauliflower rice or a veggie of your choice.

Ingredients

- Waffles
- 5 oz. of cheddar cheese
- Two large eggs
- A cup of cauliflower crumbles
- A quarter teaspoon of garlic powder
- A quarter teaspoon of onion powder
- Four tablespoons of almond flour
- Three tablespoons of parmesan cheese
- Salt and pepper
- The topping
- 4 oz. ground beef
- Four slices of chopped bacon
- Four tablespoons of sugar free barbeque sauce
- 1.5 oz. of cheddar cheese
- Salt and pepper

Nutrient intake per serving
Carbs are 3g
Fat is 29.8g
Protein is 18.8g
Calories are 354

How to prepare

1. Shred 3 oz. of cheese. You will use half for the waffle and half on top.
2. Measure out the cauliflower crumbles over a scale, or use a cup
3. Mix in half of the cheddar cheese, parmesan cheese, eggs, almond flour and spices
4. Slice the bacon thin over medium to high heat
5. As soon as the bacon is partially cooked, add in the beef.
6. Add any excess grease from the pan into the waffle mixture that you set aside
7. Immersion blend the waffle mixture into a paste that is thick
8. Add half of the mixture to the waffle iron and cook until crisp. Repeat for the second waffle

9. As the waffles cook, add in the sugar free BBQ sauce to the bacon and ground mixture of the beef.

10. Assemble the waffles together by adding half of the ground beef mixture and half of the remaining cheddar cheese to the top of the waffle

11. Broil for about two minutes until the cheese is nicely melted over the top

12. Serve immediately. You may slice up a green onion to sprinkle over the top

Bacon cheeseburger casserole (6 servings)

Ingredients

- 1 lb. ground beef
- Three slices of bacon
- Half a cup of almond flour
- 256g of cauliflower, riced
- A tablespoon of psyllium husk powder
- Half a teaspoon of garlic powder
- Half a teaspoon of onion powder
- Two tablespoons of reduced sugar ketchup
- A tablespoon of Dijon mustard
- Two tablespoons of mayonnaise
- Three large eggs
- 4 oz. cheddar cheese
- Salt and pepper

Nutrient intake per serving
Carbs are 3.6g
Fat is 35.5g
Protein is 35.2g
Calories are 478

How to prepare

1. Pre heat the oven to 350F. Put rice cauliflower in the food processor and add dry ingredients. Mix well

2. Put bacon and ground beef in food processor until crumbly and slightly past. Cook over medium to high heat. Season with salt and pepper

3. Shred the cheese as the meat cooks. Once the meat is done, mix all the ingredients in a large bowl and add half of the cheddar cheese.

4. Add eggs, mayo, ketchup and mustard to the mixture. Use a fork or hands to mix everything well

5. Press the mixture into a 9x9 baking pan lined with parchment paper. You then top with the other half of the cheddar cheese

6. Place on the top rack and bake for 25-30 minutes. For additional crisp on top, broil for around 3 minutes or until browned

7. Remove from oven and let it cool for between five to ten minutes

8. Slice and serve with additional toppings

Pumpkin pecan pie ice cream (4, one cup servings)

For extra decadence, one can add 3-4 oz. cream cheese to this recipe.

Ingredients

- Half a cup of cottage cheese
- Half a cup of pumpkin puree
- A teaspoon of pumpkin spice
- Two cups of coconut milk
- Half a teaspoon of xantham gum
- Three large egg yolks
- A third of a cup erythritol
- 20 drops of liquid stevia
- A teaspoon of maple extract
- Half a cup of pecans that are toasted & chopped
- Two tablespoons of salted butter

Nutrient intake per serving
Carbs are 4.3g
Fat is 22.3g
Protein is 6.5g
Calories are 248

How to prepare

1. Chop the toasted pecans and put on the stove with butter. Leave it over low heat until the butter turns brown. In case you don't have toasted pecans, place in a pan and toast over low heat for between 7-10 minutes

2. Place all the ingredients into a container that can accommodate the immersion blender
3. Use your immersion blender to blend all the ingredients together into a mixture that is smooth
4. Add the mixture to your ice cream machine
5. Once your butter turns brown and the pecans have soaked up some of the butter, place inside the ice cream machine
6. Follow the churning instructions as per your ice cream manufacturer's instructions

Ketogenic amaretti cookies (16 cookies)

These are delicate and sweet. Each one is soft and full of almond and fruity flavors. This recipe uses strawberry jam.

Ingredients

- A cup of almond flour
- Two tablespoons of coconut flour
- Half a teaspoon of baking powder
- A quarter teaspoon of baking powder
- A quarter teaspoon of cinnamon
- Half a teaspoon of salt
- Half a cup of erythritol
- Two large eggs
- Four tablespoons of coconut oil
- Half a teaspoon of vanilla extract
- Half a teaspoon of almond extract
- Two tablespoons of sugar free jam
- One tablespoon of organic shredded coconut

Nutrient intake per serving
Carbs are 1.2g
Fat is 7.9g
Protein is 2.4g
Calories are 86

How to prepare

1. Preheat the oven to 350F. mix all the dry ingredients and whisk
2. Add in the wet ingredients and mix well. Use a whisk or hand mixer
3. Form the cookies on a parchment paper lined baking sheet. Add an indent at the middle of each cookie using your finger or the back of a measuring spoon.
4. Bake for about 15 minutes or until the cookies turn golden or crack slightly.
5. Let the cookies cool on a wire rack and fill each indent with sugar free jam
6. Lastly, sprinkle some shredded coconut on top of each cookie
7. Dish out and serve

No bake coconut cashew bars (8 servings)

These bars are easy to make and can be frozen or refrigerated depending on what you need.

Ingredients

- A cup of almond flour
- A quarter cup of melted butter
- A quarter cup of sugar free maple syrup
- A teaspoon of cinnamon
- A pinch of salt
- Half a cup of cashews
- A quarter cup of shredded coconut

Nutrient intake per serving
Carbs are 4g
Fat is 17.6g
Protein is 4g
Calories are 189

How to prepare

1. Mix the melted butter and almond flour in a large bowl
2. Add cinnamon, salt and sugar free maple syrup and mix properly
3. You then add the shredded coconut and mix again
4. Roughly chop half a cup of cashews whether raw or roasted. Add to the coconut cashew bar dough. Mix well

5. Line a baking dish with parchment paper and spread the coconut cashew bar dough in an even layer. You can add some more shredded coconut and cinnamon on top
6. Place them in the refrigerator and chill for at least two hours. However, overnight is recommended. As soon as they are chilled, slice them into bars.
7. Serve and enjoy!

Ketogenic chocolate covered macaroons (12 macaroons)

These macaroons are sweet with a nice coconut, almond and chocolate flavor.

Ingredients

- A cup of unsweetened shredded coconut
- A large white egg
- A quarter cup of erythritol
- Half a teaspoon of almond extract
- A pinch of salt
- 20 grams of sugar free chocolate
- Two tablespoons of coconut oil

Nutrient intake per serving
Carbs are 1g
Fat is 7.3g
Protein is 1g
Calories are 73

How to prepare

1. Preheat the oven to 350F and spread a cup of shredded and unsweetened coconut into a thin layer on a parchment paper lined baking sheet. As soon as the oven is hot enough, place the coconut in to toast up a little for about five minutes.
2. As the coconut toasts, beat the egg white until it's foamy
3. Add the erythritol and a pinch of salt as you continue to mix.
4. You then add the almond extract for a twist on normal coconut macaroons.
5. Once the coconut flakes have toasted and cooled, add them in and fold everything together

6. Use an ice cream scoop or your hands to tightly pack little balls of macaroon batter and gently place them on a parchment paper lined baking sheet. Bake until they are golden. This should take around 15 minutes

7. As they bake, make the chocolate drizzle by melting coconut oil and the sugar free chocolate. Continuously stir to make sure the chocolate doesn't burn

8. When the macaroons are out of the oven

9. Drizzle your chocolate over each one of them.

Ketogenic chocolate peanut butter tarts(4 servings)

Ingredients

- Crust
- A quarter cup of flaxseeds
- Two tablespoons of almond flour
- A tablespoon of erythritol
- A large egg white
- Top layer
- A medium avocado
- Four tablespoons of cocoa powder
- A quarter cup of erythritol
- Half a teaspoon of vanilla extract
- Half a teaspoon of cinnamon
- Two tablespoons of heavy cream
- Middle layer
- Four tablespoons of peanut butter
- Two tablespoons of butter

Nutrient intake per serving
Carbs are 3.9g
Fat is 26.8g
Protein is 9.8g
Calories are 305

How to prepare

1. Preheat the oven to 350F. Make your crust by grinding up a quarter cup of flaxseeds until they are finely ground.
2. Add the rest of the crust ingredients to the ground flaxseeds.
3. Blend until well mixed
4. Press the crust mixture into the tart pans and up the sides. Bake for about 8 minutes until set
5. As the crust bakes, prepare the top layer by mixing all the ingredients in a blender and blend until smooth and creamy
6. After removing the crusts from the oven, let them cool as you prepare your peanut butter layer. Melt the peanut butter and butter in the microwave or a small pan over the stove until well mixed and soft
7. Pour the melted layer of peanut butter onto the tart crusts and place in the fridge for half an hour until set
8. As soon as the top of the peanut butter layer is set, add the chocolate avocado layer on top. Smooth it out and refrigerate for an hour.
9. Slice, serve and enjoy

In this chapter I will list down a few ketogenic bodybuilding meal plans for biological Men and Woman.

Men

Breakfast

- Four eggs
- An ounce of cheddar cheese
- Four bacon slices

Nutrient intake per serving
Carbs are 2g
Fat is 36.3g
Protein is 44.2g
Calories are 521

Pre Workout Shake

- A scoop of whey
- 250ml of unsweetened almond milk
- Two tablespoons of peanut butter

Nutrient intake per serving
Carbs are 9.3g
Fat is 18.6g
Protein is 31g
Calories are 318

Lunch

- 200g of chicken breast trimmed of fat / 200g turkey breasts/ 220g tilapia
- Side salad(60g spinach, half a carrot, half a cucumber and a stalk of celery
- 50g avocado
- Two tablespoons of balsamic vinegar
- A tablespoon of olive oil

Nutrient intake per serving
Carbs are 14.3g
Fat is 26.7g
Protein is 49.8g
Calories are 503

Men

Dinner

- 150g veggies
- A tablespoon of butter

Nutrient intake per serving

Carbs are 9.9g

Fat is 15g

Protein is 55.2g

Calories are 389

Snack

- 200g of 4% cottage cheese
- 20 almonds or peanuts

Nutrient intake per serving

Carbs are 14.5g

Fat is 19.7g

Protein is 23.6g

Calories are 324

Women

Breakfast

- Two eggs
- An ounce of cheddar cheese
- Three bacon slices

Nutrient intake per serving

Carbs are 1.2g

Fat is 24.6g

Protein is 28.6g

Calories are 347

Post Workout Shake

- A scoop of whey
- A cup of unsweetened almond milk
- A cup of strawberries/almond butter

Nutrient intake per serving

Carbs are 17g

Fat is 10.6g

Protein is 27g

Calories are 268

Women

Lunch

- 7 ounces of chicken breasts trimmed of fat
- Salad(two cups of spinach, half a carrot, half a cucumber and half a tomato)
- Two ounces of feta cheese
- Two tablespoons of balsamic vinegar
- A tablespoon of olive oil

Nutrient intake per serving
Carbs are 15.8g
Fat is 21.1g
Protein is 51.1g
Calories are 462

Snack

- 20 almonds or peanuts

Nutrient intake per serving
Carbs are 5.2g
Fat is 12g
Protein is 5.1g
Calories are 139

Dinner

- 7 ounces sirloin trimmed of fat
- 6 ounces veggies
- A tablespoon of butter

Nutrient intake per serving
Carbs are 12.2g
Fat is 19.9g
Protein is 49.6g
Calories are 426

The right way of cooking vegetables

There are cooking methods that preserve nutrients in veggies while others can
destroy them.

Limit the water

When veggies are cooked in water, they lose nutrients. To retain the nutrients, cook
veggies in as little water as possible for the minimal amount of time. Furthermore,
steaming and microwaving also lead to less loss of nutrients.

Use some fat

Nutrients like beta carotene, vitamin D and K are fat soluble and can only get into
the blood stream with some fat.

Wash before cutting

Cutting veggies allows the escape of nutrients. By washing prior to cutting, nutrients
will safely remain in the cell walls.

Keep the vegetable peels on if possible

Foods to avoid with the ketogenic diet

Any foods that are high in carbohydrates should be limited. One should cut down
on sugary foods, grains or starches, fruits, beans, root veggies and tubers, low fat
diets, selected sauces, booze and sugar free diets.

French fries and potato chips

They contain a lot of calories and one can consume a lot of them. Consumption of
fries and potato chips is connected to gaining of weight. A study revealed that these
foods contribute to gaining of weight than any other food. Furthermore, baked,
roasted or froes potatoes contain cancer causing ingredients. It is advisable to eat
plain, boiled potatoes.

French fries and potato chips are fattening and unhealthy.

Drinks that are sugary

Beverages like soda are one of the unhealthiest foods on earth. They are strongly linked to gaining of weight and are detrimental to one's health if taken in excess. Liquid calories do not make you feel satisfied and you will add these calories on top of your normal intake. If you want to lose weight, steer clear of these drinks.

White bread

It is highly refined and contains lots of added sugars. It ranks high on the glycemic index and can raise levels of sugar. A study revealed that eating two slices of white bread in a day was linked to a greater risk of adding weight and being obese. Bread that is made from very fine flour can raise sugar levels and cause one to overeat.

Candy bars

They are quite unhealthy because they stack a lot of sugar, added oils and refined flour. Furthermore, they are high in calories and low in nutritive value. An average candy bar contains an average of 250 calories. If you crave for snacks, eat a fruit or nuts.

Most fruit juices

Many of the fruit juices found in stores have very little similarity to the whole fruit. They are highly processed and contain a lot of sugar. They contain as much sugar as soda or even more. These juices also contain no fibers and they will not have the same effect as real fruits.

Pastries and cakes

They have unhealthy ingredients such as added sugar and refined flour. Furthermore, they also contain artificial Trans- fats which are very harmful and connected to several diseases. Additionally, they are less satisfying and you will feel hungry very fast after eating them.

Alcohol

It provides more calories than carbohydrates and protein. Consumption of alcohol in moderation is okay; however, heavy drinking is linked to increased gaining of weight. Beer causes gaining of weight.

Ice cream

This is quite unhealthy, high in calories and loaded with sugar. Think about making your own ice cream using less sugar and healthier ingredients like yogurt and fruit. Additionally, serve yourself small portions so as to avoid eating too much.

Pizza

Ones that are made commercially are very unhealthy. They contain high calories and often contain unhealthy ingredients such as refined flour and meat that is processed. It is better to make pizzas at home because they are healthier.

Coffee drinks with high calories

They are loaded with empty calories that can be the same as a whole meal. Plain, black coffee is very healthy and can aid in fat burning. However, such drinks have artificial ingredients that are very unhealthy and fattening.

Foods with a lot of added sugar

Examples are sugary breakfast cereals and flavored yogurt.

Soy sauce

Even though it is low on calories, it has high sodium content that can make you bloated and increase your chances of getting hypertension.

Tropical fruits

There are some to avoid if you want to lose weight. Take limited mangoes and ripe pineapples because they contain a lot of sugar.

Foods to eat

You should consume plenty of meat, fatty fish, eggs, butter and cream, cheese, nuts and seeds, healthy oils, avocados, low carb veggies and condiments.

Healthy ketogenic diets

In case you feel like eating something between meals, the following are advised:

- Fatty fish or meat
- Cheese
- A handful of nuts
- Cheese with olives
- 1-2 hard-boiled eggs
- 90% dark chocolate

Great snacks for a ketogenic diet include pieces of meat, cheese, olives and dark chocolate.

Tips for eating out on a ketogenic diet

Several restaurants offer some kind of meat or fish, or dishes that are fish based. You can order this and replace foods containing high carbs with veggies. Meals that are egg based are also a good idea.

In short, when eating out, choose meat, fish or egg based foods. Also order extra vegetables rather than carbohydrates or starch.

Supplements for a ketogenic diet

Even though taking of supplements is not needed, some could prove helpful.

MCT oil - it is added to drinks or yogurt. It gives energy and aids in the increment of ketone levels.

Minerals - added salt and other minerals are useful when beginning the diet. This is because of the alterations in mineral and water balance.

Caffeine - can provide energy, aid in losing fat and enhance performance.

Exogenous ketones - this can help raise the levels of ketones in your body.

Creatine - this supplement has several benefits for one's health and performance. It is advisable if one combines ketogenic diets with exercise.

Whey - this increases the intake of daily protein.

Sources of protein for the vegan keto diet

- Tofu
- Pumpkin seed
- Almond
- Walnut
- Pecan
- Coconut
- Low carb veggies
- Lettuce
- Bok choy
- Beet greens
- Spinach
- Asparagus
- Collard greens
- Cucumber
- Broccoli
- Low carb fruits
- Lemon juice
- Rhubarb
- Lime juice
- Raspberries
- Strawberries

It is also important for you to know that veggies have more carbs as compared to sources of meat. And since vegans mostly rely on increased amounts of veggies and fruits, on should be careful to limit the carbs intake. It does not matter whether you are a vegan or carnivore because ketosis is a normal state that your body goes through.

Unhealthy ways of losing weight

Zero calorie diet
Our bodies require fat, healthy fats that assist in burning fat.

Drugs and pills
There is no magic pill that helps one to shed weight. Drugs such as cocaine and heroin are usually used for losing weight. However, in the long run, they damage the heart as well as the brain. Supplements that aid in weight loss must be coupled with healthy eating and exercise.

Skipping meals
It may appear to make sense but it is harmful and unhealthy. A person's metabolism increases after eating and by missing meals, you slow down the metabolism and the result could be gaining of weight.

Inducing vomiting
This is harmful to one's health. This happens because of underlying psychological effects on someone. Vomiting is a symptom or leads to bulimia. Furthermore, it will also increase the craving for foods that are not healthy. Vomiting creates an illusion that the hunger craving is satisfied by consumption of food, however, you lose calories by vomiting.

Use of laxatives
Too much use of laxatives using pills, powders and teas to induce weight loss is not new. If used continuously, this will make the digestive system weak and cause complications of the abdomen.

Smoking

This is another way people use to cut appetite. It sends signals to the brain, this increase the rate of metabolism and kills hunger. Chronic smokers skip meals regularly. This method causes long term damage to the body by making it weak and more vulnerable to infections and ailments.

Fasting in excess

Excessive fasting induces insomnia, anxiety and loss of fertility.

CONCLUSION

I want to thank you and congratulate you for downloading and reading this book, Ketogenic Diet for Beginners.

This book has surely offered you the proven steps and strategies on how to get into a ketogenic diet that is healthy and beneficial to your health. The Ketogenic diet is one of the most popular diets in the world of weight loss right now for many reasons.

Thousands have enjoyed the many health benefits including lower blood pressure, lower cholesterol, more energy, clearer thinking, and of course weight loss. Many also believe and follow the ketogenic diet to fight cancer as well.

The ketogenic diet allows you to eat real foods, the ones you are already used to eating, and you will still lose the weight you want to lose. Using proven methods to help your body and metabolism work together, you will lose weight and build muscles in your sleep!

This book has taught you all about the Ketogenic Diet basics and it is now time to put what you have read into practice. This book has also offered you the recipes, benefits and proven ways of benefitting from the Ketogenic diet. It details the health benefits of this diet and ways of starting and maintaining it.

Thank you again for downloading this book!

I hope this book was able to help you to eat and live healthy by following the Ketogenic diet. The next step is to follow the instructions and stick to a healthy diet for all round wellness.